INTRO to
BIOHACKING

Be Smarter, Stronger, and Happier

Ari R. Meisel

CONTENTS

INTRO

what is biohacking?

Welcome to the fascinating, ever changing, and always adapting world of biohacking. My name is Ari Meisel, and I've created this study to help you harness the cooperative power of mind, body, and spirit in order to generate a more fulfilling, healthier, and more productive life.

In this text, we'll cover a variety of biohacking topics, like the brain, sleep, nutrition, supplementation, and much more. We'll learn how these aspects of physical, mental, and spiritual health interact with one another. We'll cover basic tips, tricks, or "hacks" that one can perform to improve overall bodily function. After reading, you'll be armed with several useful strategies for improving your own well-being, and you'll be well on your way to hacking the often complicated workings of the body to generate a healthier you.

So, what exactly is biohacking? Don't worry; it has nothing to do with separating limbs from the body or performing dangerous self-surgeries. The word "hack" is used to denote any improvised solution. Doing something out of the ordinary in a way that works for you is a hack. With biohacking, we're essentially hacking our own bodies, creating unique, out of the ordinary solutions for common health problems like exhaustion, weight gain, poor nutrition, difficulty concentrating, and much more.

As humans, we have three essential fields of health: bodily health, mental health, and spiritual health. Every common ailment or health struggle can generally fall into one of these categories. Similarly, every solution to these problems can also fit within these groups. With this biohacking guide, you'll discover ways to improve overall health by cheating the system and using unconventional tactics, surprising solutions, and out of the ordinary habits in areas like the brain, sleep, nutrition, supplementation, fitness, and more.

Now, in any field of study, there are numerous subtopics, additional worlds of information, and the potential for limitless learning and understanding. The world of biohacking is no different. To cover every aspect of every topic would be, in a word, overwhelming. Sure, we could visit each and every intricacy of a topic like the brain, dissect all of the latest scientific information, and work to become brain experts, but that process could and would take a lifetime.

To make the subject of biohacking a little more practical and palatable, I've included three basic strategies in every category. These three basic strategies will work for everyone; they are strategies that every person should adopt because they will lead to healthy improvements. In each category, I'll also provide one advanced strategy. For individuals looking for an additional health leap, these advanced strategies are a great way to seek out even greater biological improvements.

What Makes Me a Biohacker?

In 2007, I was diagnosed with Crohn's Disease, a painful, embarrassing, and ultimately incurable condition. Overweight, wracked with pain, subjected to extensive testing, bloodwork, and multiple colonoscopies, my doctors delivered the devastating news: both my small and large intestines, as well as my stomach, had been devastated by severe Crohn's.

This complicated ailment led to other bodily malfunctions. My liver health began to suffer. I was diagnosed with kidney stones. My body, once healthy and vibrant, was beginning to shut down, essentially "giving up" due to an inordinate number of health issues. When my body started giving up, my mind was quick to follow. I had difficulty rolling out of bed in the morning; I was required to take sixteen different medications that affected my mood, disposition, and physical health. Medications led to hair loss, extreme nausea, and dangerous emotional swings.

My Crohn's Disease affected, not just my physical health, but my relationships, as well. Embarrassment of my symptoms, prolonged hospital stays, and emotional chaos was preventing me from engaging in healthy, productive relationships. It started with Crohn's. It led to total, annihilating chaos. My physical, mental, and spiritual health felt like they were swirling into a void.

A change was necessary. My biohacking journey started with yoga and a nutritional overhaul. I started practicing relaxation and calming techniques through meditation. I stripped my diet of everything but vegetarian-approved dishes, replaced butter with olive oil, and started eating quinoa and kale rather than steaks and French fries. I also began experimenting with vitamins and other forms of supplementation.

In addition to diet changes, I began seeking information about the human body and overall wellness. I became an EMT and a yoga instructor and started dabbling in extreme endurance sports. Beating my disease wasn't enough; I needed to crush it into submission and let my body know that these health issues were not going to dictate my future.

After years of training, self-education, commitment to dietary changes, and deciding, every day, to make overall health my primary goal, I went back for a scheduled visit with my physician. The usual battery of tests revealed something amazing: my incurable Crohn's Disease had disappeared. There was no evidence of inflammation anywhere in my body. I had, essentially, hacked my own body and, through a few significant changes, altered the course of my future.

I'm a biohacker.

Today, I'm stronger than I was before my diagnosis, and I attribute this change to biohacking. I am not an exception to the rule. I believe, firmly, that everyone can achieve life-altering results like mine. I've made it my mission to share my journey, my processes, and my biohacking techniques with the world.

You may be reading this because you're experiencing your own assortment of overwhelming health issues. You may feel like you're at the end of your own rope. Your future may appear hopelessly bleak. I am here to tell you that biohacking can create positive, dramatic, and sustainable change in your life.

It starts with a first step. Are you ready to take yours?

ONE

fitness

P hysical fitness is probably the one area of overall health that most people want to improve in their own lives. We live in a world where physical fitness is declining at an alarming rate. Obesity is becoming the norm rather than an exception. Ailing fitness is a slippery slope, and it can lead to dangerous health issues like diabetes, heart disease, and even premature death.

If you want to use biohacking to improve your fitness levels, the three basic improvement areas are: strength, conditioning, and mobility. Boosting these three aspects of physical fitness will create dramatic results in your own body. At the end of this section, you'll also find an advanced tip to help you take your fitness journey to the next level.

Strength

Depending on what you want to achieve, there are many different directions you can go to improve physical strength. There are those who want to achieve maximum strength capabilities and push their bodies to the very limits of human achievement. Most people don't want their biceps to be bigger around than a tree trunk, so the strength conditioning we're talking about here is just a matter of maintaining a healthy body by improving balance, coordination, and functional movement.

If this is your goal, then less is actually more as far as strength conditioning is concerned. Visiting the gym every day, running for miles and miles on the treadmill, and lifting weights every other day is really unnecessary. For general health and improved strength and functionality, a single, effective, common exercise is all you need.

This exercise is called "The Manmaker."

For this exercise, you can start with no weight and progress to using dumbbells or kettle bells. This is a series exercise, which means that one complete repetition of the exercise involves a few different parts completed in quick succession. Here's how to do The Manmaker.

1. Start in a standing position with your feet shoulder-width apart. If you're using weights, you can hold them in your hands or place them directly in front of your feet.
2. Perform a single push-up.
3. Use your right arm to perform a single-arm row with your dumbbell or kettle bell while remaining in push-up position.
4. Perform another single push-up.
5. Use your left arm this time to perform another single-arm row, and return to a push-up position.
6. Bring your legs forward between your arms until you reach a squat position.
7. Squat-Clean the dumbbells or kettle bells. This is an important part of The Manmaker. A "Clean" involves simply lifting a weight from the floor to your shoulders. In a Squat-Clean, you utilize an explosive motion to pull the weight off the floor onto your shoulders while receiving the weight in a squatted position. It is very important that you end with your hips below your knees. In other words, your squat should be deep, your thighs lowered beyond parallel to the floor.
8. Stand and push-press the weights fully over your head.

Those eight steps represent one Manmaker repetition. Your goal, depending on the weight that you use, should be about three sets of three Manmaker repetitions. This exercise should only take you about ten minutes, and you'll achieve incredible strength results with just this one exercise.

Start at a weight and pace that is challenging but not excessive. As your body strengthens, increase the weights used, the number of repetitions, or the number of sets performed. The Manmaker is a great biohack for improving strength and fitness.

Conditioning

Conditioning is essentially your body's cardiovascular capacity or the rate at which your heart and lungs are able to use and process oxygen in order to keep muscles working at an accelerated rate. To improve conditioning, most people think they have to start a long-distance running or cycling regimen. Newcomers to conditioning training may jump on a treadmill and run at a steady, average pace for as long as they can.

The truth is this isn't the most effective way to improve conditioning. Interval training, the process of performing high intensity cardio activities for short periods of time, is a much more effective way of improving cardiovascular health. Tabata training, a high intensity interval workout created by a Japanese physician, is one of the simplest, most effective training methods.

Tabata training involves 20 seconds of very intense exercise followed by 10 seconds of complete rest, which forms one Tabata interval. A complete Tabata training routine consists of eight interval repetitions. Have you done the math, yet? That adds up to only four minutes of total workout time. This might seem too good to be true, but correct Tabata training will have you drenched in sweat long before you finish.

What exercises can you do during the 20 seconds of high intensity training? Just about anything. Sprints, squats, Jumping Jacks, swimming sprints, and other full-body, high intensity exercises are all effective.

During the 20 seconds of active exercises, you should push your body as hard and fast as possible. Extensive tests and studies have shown that this incredibly brief yet intense training style is as effective, or even more effective, than an hour of steady, paced cardio training.

One hour of cardio or four minutes of Tabata interval training? That's an easy choice and a great biohack to improve your conditioning and overall fitness levels.

Mobility

Mobility is one aspect of overall fitness that is often neglected and overlooked. With our on-the-go lifestyles, we rarely take the time to heal our ligaments, connective tissue, posture, and other important parts of physical health. Resting by sitting or lying down really isn't enough; instead, mobility-improving exercises are needed to restore the body and give it a chance to recuperate. This is especially true for individuals with stressful, active, or fast-paced lifestyles.

Yoga is a great mobility-improving activity. Yoga motions include twisting, stretching, and even strength exercises. Yoga also includes a meditative aspect, which improves mental and spiritual health along with physical health. The persistent practice of yoga will help you complete everyday tasks with greater ease and efficiency.

Even with mountains of research and supportive science, many people still balk at the idea of joining a yoga class. They may be embarrassed, uncomfortable, consider yoga too feminine or too new-age, or simply fail to recognize the healing and health-improving benefits of this ancient practice. "Yoga? It's not for me," you may have said in the past. It's time to change our collective opinion of yoga: it is for everybody. Including you.

Here's a yoga biohack that you can use to improve mobility. If you don't want to join a class or learn the art of yoga in front of a crowd, download the Yoga Studio application to a smart phone or tablet. Within the app, you can download one or several different, customizable yoga routines to perform in the comfort of your own home. The app allows you to customize the length of the routine, so you can fit in a quick yoga session whenever you have free time. Helpful, guided videos will show you exactly how to perform the movements correctly and safely.

Advanced

What if you're ready to take your fitness biohacking to the next level? If you've used the above steps to improve your strength, conditioning, and mobility, but you're craving an additional challenge, there is a wealth of information available to help you achieve your fitness goals. Most people, when they reach a certain level of physical fitness, develop their own goal ideas. You may, for example, want to deadlift 500 pounds, run a marathon, or complete a Triathlon event. These are all great goals, and they are very achievable. You can find helpful tips online or from a personal trainer to help you achieve those goals.

What if, though, you don't have a goal in mind? If you're searching for a new fitness achievement, allow me to introduce you to the world of Krav Maga. Developed by the Israeli military, Krav Maga is a form of self-defense and hand-to-hand combat that relies on several different techniques including boxing, wrestling, and even Judo.

This is a great biohack because everyone can benefit from some basic knowledge in self-defense. Learning Martial Arts can help with the development of self-confidence. It can help you learn about the capabilities and limitations of your own body. Most importantly, though, it can help with stress management. Krav Maga is a full-contact version of Martial Arts training. Repeatedly taking a hit during training might sound scary and horrible, but it helps the body to develop resilience. This resilience can be incredibly helpful in stressful situations. Your body will have learned to bounce back from Krav Maga contact, and this ability translates to everyday life situations. You're tougher and stronger than you think, and Krav Maga can help you realize that truth.

TWO

brain

Ah, the brain: that mysterious, powerful, seemingly limitless organ nestled beneath half an inch of bone. The human brain is truly remarkable. Modern democracy, lasting works of art, social developments and improvements, the discoveries of the cosmos, and the technological inventions of our age have all been developed and cultivated within a lumpy, wrinkled human organ. Our brains have incredible potential, and biohacking can help to unlock this potential.

This chapter discusses biohacking techniques for brain improvement, increased resilience, and even brain expansion. At the end, I've included an advanced brain biohacking technique that you can use to further develop your body's most important organ.

Improvement

When it comes to improving cognitive function and performance, the science of neuroplasticity basically suggests that brain function can be improved by working the brain in much the same way as one would work out a muscle in another part of the body. You can perform arm curls that challenge and stretch the biceps in order to increase muscle size and performance ability. The muscle is pushed to its limit, and after it is given the chance to recover it's revealed to be bigger and stronger than it was before.

By "working out" the brain, you can achieve similar effects and see dramatic brain function improvement over time. How, though, does one "work out" the brain? There are no weight lifting techniques that you can use to stretch or challenge this organ. Instead, you can use brain-training games to push the brain's current capacity and see overall improvement.

Brainturk.com is a free, brain-training website that is a great alternative to some of the paid brain strengthening applications. Within the site, you'll find a few different game categories. Agility, for example, improves the brain's ability to think and adapt quickly. Other games improve memory, recall, problem solving, and fluid intelligence. Games that use and challenge different intelligence types or different aspects of the brain's function will provide more positive effects.

Training your brain doesn't require a huge investment of time or energy. Even playing one single brain game for five minutes each day will result in dramatic improvements to overall brain function.

Resilience

Brain resilience refers to the brain's ability to cognitively change autonomic nervous system functions. Normally, things like heart rate and breathing rate are independent of our conscious brain function. You don't have to consciously decide to make your heart beat; your body just manages this job on its own. This means, though, that these functions can be negatively affected by things like stress in our lives. When you encounter a stressful situation, your heart rate speeds up. Brain resilience, then, is the ability to supersede this autonomic response and intentionally calm your body. With practice, you can do this even in the face of extreme stress.

Meditation is the most common method of improving brain resilience, but it can be frustrating for many people because it requires time, patience, and incredible control over mental functions. If you don't have time to master meditation in order to improve your brain's resilience, you can achieve the same effects in a fraction of the time by using a Heart Rate Variability app. Heart Rate Variability is a system of measure that has been around for quite awhile, and it's a great method for determining how your breathing rate, heart rate, and other autonomic nervous system functions respond to stress and other life events.

Stress Doctor from Azumio is a great smartphone application that will measure your heart rate and allow you to visualize your autonomic functions while performing relaxation techniques. To use the application, you simply place your fingertip over the camera of your smartphone. Immediately, the app begins measuring your heart rate and displaying it as a constantly changing line graph. By visualizing your heart rate and seeing your stress as a visual graphic rather than simply perceiving it internally, you can practice brain resilience.
Breathing in and out, thinking of positive thoughts and ideas, and even changing your posture or environment will result in heart changes that you can visualize.

Improving brain resilience can lead to reduced stress, greater control over one's life circumstances, better sleep, and overall improved health. Using a Heart Rate Variability app is a biohack with incredible potential.

Expansion

Expanding the brain's power by learning new things is an important part of improving brain health. You've probably heard the urban legend that every time a new idea is learned, a new wrinkle appears in the brain. That's not entirely true, but learning new things does create new neural connections within our brain. Constantly creating new neural connections and expanding the brain's potential will help to improve overall function and maintain brain vitality.

The problem is, learning new things takes time and effort. That's why many people turn to accelerated learning software. It can be difficult, though, to find software that effectively expands the brain and allows for knowledge retention. For example, there is an abundance of learning software available for people who wish to learn a new language. This software, though, requires hours of effort, and many people discover that they have difficulty retaining the information covered in the lessons.

When it comes to accelerated learning, there are a variety of different methods that can be used. Repetition, the use of flash cards, speaking aloud, or writing are all learning methods with scientific research to back them up. Not all methods work for all people, however.

BrainScape.com uses a method known as Spaced Repetition, which is one of the most effective accelerated learning techniques. The algorithm used by BrainScape is finely tuned to the individual doing the learning, which allows it to determine the precise amount of space to place between repetitions of information. This space improves knowledge retention and increases brain expansion.

Users can answer questions and, if the question is answered correctly, users can tell the program how confidently they answered the question. If you get lucky with a guess, you can tell BrainScape to continue giving you that question until you know the answer by heart. The amount of information and knowledge contained at BrainScape.com is incredible. There are programs for learning languages, geography, history, music theory, sports history, and much more. Students can also use AP Exam prep courses to brush up on school subjects and improve exam performance.

Advanced

For advanced brain performance biohacking, you might want to consider the growing field of brain function supplementation. The movie Limitless explored this controversial subject in a very engaging way. While the little miracle pill in this film was entirely fictional, there are some prescription medications that have been proven to improve brain function dramatically and immediately.

Taking a prescription brain booster, though, is controversial and may have unexplored health effects. Instead, a positive biohack that can help you improve brain function can be found at Onnit.com. This reputable producer of supplements has an all-natural, herbal brain-boosting supplement called Alpha BRAIN. This supplement is well-supported by scientific research and clinical testing. It includes naturally occurring ingredients like Alpha GPC, Oat Straw, Vitamin B, and much more.

One interesting ingredient is Bacopa: an Ayurvedic brain nutrient. Ayurvedic treatments are not discussed prominently in health circles, but there are several PubMed studies that have revealed this ingredient to have powerful brain-boosting effects.

If you are interested in supplementation to improve brain function, it is crucial that you use consistent self-testing to evaluate the efficacy of whatever supplement you are taking. You can use some of the same websites, applications, and software we've discussed earlier to test your brain's ability before and after taking a specific supplement. By measuring and recording your results, you'll figure out what supplements have the most positive, measurable effect on your overall cognitive power.

THREE

sleep

Sleep is, without a doubt, one of the most important parts of overall health. Inadequate sleep can lead to weight gain, memory problems, heart disease, increased chances for a stroke or heart attack, high blood pressure, reduced cognitive function, decreased ability to operate a vehicle, and much more.

Even with all of the overwhelming evidence supporting the importance of sleep in determining overall health, we still are seeing an increasing number of sleep problems and decreasing total hours of sleep per person each night. Our hectic lifestyles, demanding job schedules, and even our televisions and smart phones may be contributing to our sleeplessness.

Biohacking is a great way to improve your sleeping habits and get the most positive effects from a single night's sleep. Biohacking tactics like sleep timing and environment will help to reduce sleeplessness. If you're ready to get the best night's sleep of your life, press forward and adopt some of these biohacking habits.

Timing

Have you ever woken up from a beautiful, comfortable, eight-hour night of sleep expecting to feel rejuvenated and invigorated only to discover that you feel groggy and cranky? Ever experienced that moment where your alarm goes off and it feels like you just laid your head down a few minutes ago? It's a common problem, and it's actually a simple fix.

More and more studies are showing that the length of sleep time is not nearly as important as the period of the sleep cycle during which you awake. During a single night's sleep, the human body goes through several stages of wakefulness. REM Sleep, or Rapid Eye Movement Sleep, is a light stage of sleeping. This is the stage during which dreams occur, and it is characterized by the rapid motion of the eyes beneath the eyelids. REM Sleep alternates with four different stages of deep sleep. If an alarm clock starts ringing while your body is going through a deep stage of sleep, you'll wake up groggy and frustrated.

How can you prevent yourself from being jolted from deep sleep by your alarm clock? Sleepyti.me is an online sleep calculator that will tell you when to head to bed in order to wake up feeling rested at a specific time. This calculator is based on an average sleep cycle length of 90 minutes. To use the calculator, enter the time you need to wake up. Sleepyti.me will use the 90-minute sleep cycle to give you four different options for when to go to sleep.

You should also take note of how long, on average, it takes you to fall asleep. The human average is about fourteen minutes, so this time should be taken into account when determining when to lie down for the night.

Environment

In today's modern world, we are constantly surrounded by lights. Street lights, headlights, computer screens, televisions, and smartphone screens produce blue-spectrum light. This spectrum of light tricks the body into thinking that the sun is still up. Our bodies are very attuned to the rise and fall of the sun, and when the sun sets in an environment without artificial light, a hormone called Melatonin is produced. Melatonin creates that sleepy feeling, and it tells us that it's time for bed.

When we're surrounded by artificial blue-spectrum light, though, our bodies get confused. Studies have shown that excessive screen viewing, especially at night, can prevent the production of Melatonin. It's no wonder, then, that we have trouble falling asleep; our bodies don't know that it's nighttime!

Some people counteract this effect by taking Melatonin supplements before bedtime, but this is really treating the symptom not the problem. We could go totally crazy and eliminate electronic device usage a full hour before bedtime, but who is going to really have the discipline required to turn off the TV, shut down the computer, and put away the iPhone before bed? No one.

Here's a biohacking solution that will regulate your body's Melatonin production without requiring you to abstain from your favorite shows or your beloved device: Blue Blocking Sunglasses. For just $10, you can buy a pair of sunglasses that completely block blue-spectrum light. Wearing these sunglasses an hour before bedtime will result in better sleep the very first night you use them. You can watch television, browse your favorite websites, or check out social media without bombarding your brain with confusing blue-spectrum light waves.

Clear

Our sleep cycling and our nighttime routines can have a dramatic effect on sleep quality, but one of the biggest factors that impairs healthy sleep is actually a product of our environment. Sleep is the body's chance to recharge its batteries. It is a natural function that almost all animals perform. During sleep, the body repairs organ and tissue damage, recovers from fatigue and exertion, and eliminates toxins from the body. After successfully completing this recovery process, the body signals to the brain that it is time to wake up. You, then, open your eyes and feel rejuvenated and ready to start a new day.

What happens, though, if the body is so loaded down with toxins and impurities that it cannot repair itself in a single night? When the body works all night long to remove toxins and regenerate, you wake up in the morning feeling groggy and tired. Your body is essentially saying, "I need more time! I'm not done healing yet!"

So, here's a great biohack that you can use to have a healthier, more fulfilling night's sleep. By taking a Liposomal Glutathione supplement, you can help your body remove dangerous toxins. Glutathione is naturally found in the body. In fact, it's the substance that our body relies on most to flush out environmental toxins. By supplementing with additional oxidized Glutathione, you'll give your body an extra toxin-beating boost.

Some people take charcoal supplements because of their toxin-eliminating effects. Charcoal was often prescribed to patients with nausea or upset stomach, especially after eating something toxic or unhealthy. Charcoal, though, is only effective when the toxin was consumed recently. For deep-set toxins in the bloodstream, tissue, and organs, Glutathione is the best solution.

Advanced

You've adjusted your sleep time to coordinate with your sleep cycles. You've eliminated excessive blue-spectrum light pollution from your evening routine in order to encourage the body to generate healthy levels of Melatonin. Finally, you've helped the body to flush out toxins with supplements that improve sleep's effectiveness.

Now, you're ready to take your night of sleep to the next level. The Remee Lucid Dreaming sleep mask is a fascinating, slightly off-the-wall product that is generating a lot of consumer interest. Lucid Dreaming is a practice wherein an individual can remain lucid while dreaming during sleep.

Typically, a dream is just a random upchuck of information in the brain. There is very little control over a dream's content, which is why many people jump from location to location or plop down in the middle of an out-of-control situation during their dreams. Lucid Dreaming, on the other hand, allows the dreamer to control his or her own dream.

The Remee Lucid Dreaming sleep mask has LED lights that can flash in a specific, individualized pattern during sleep. Once you've fallen asleep, the LED lights will begin flashing in colors and patterns that you have chosen. So, if you're dreaming of staring out at the Caribbean Sea and you suddenly see flashing red lights over the water, your dream self will recognize that you are experiencing a dream, and you can begin to control your environment or activities. Always wanted to fly? This mask might help you do that in your dreams.

Lucid Dreaming isn't just fun and games, however. There have been studies suggesting that Lucid Dreaming may be a safe and effective way for people to face their fears or shortcomings. If you're afraid of public speaking, for example, you can enter into a public speaking environment during your dream. You will know that the event is not really happening, but you will still be able to participate in a very realistic public speaking experience.

We spend a third of our lives sleeping. By practicing Lucid Dreaming, you can turn this "wasted" time into productive, beneficial growth and development.

FOUR

nutrition

Nutrition is, far and away, the most crucial element of overall, top to bottom healthy living. Unfortunately, it's also the aspect of physical, mental, and spiritual health that is most often neglected. Our lives are hectic, and it's tempting to grab the quickest and most convenient food source you can find while you rush from home to work to school to all of the other commitments placing demands on your day.

It's helpful sometimes to think of the human body as the most complex and sophisticated machine on the planet. That's really all the body is: a beautifully functioning, harmonious machine of interworking parts. If you continually filled your automobile with low quality fuel, choked the engine with gunky oil, and never lifted the hood to see how the parts were functioning, how long could you expect that vehicle to run smoothly and reliably? The answer is obvious: not very long at all.

The same is true for the human body. When your main fuel sources come from chemically processed, nutrient-free, worthless food items, it should come as no surprise when bodily processes start shutting down, organs stop functioning correctly, and adverse symptoms start popping up.

Overhauling your diet can seem like a daunting task. We know that we need to eat better, but we don't know how to get started. We're surrounded by conflicting nutritional information from diet "experts," confusing labels on our favorite foods that make the food item sound healthy, and tempting, delicious snacks that make our mouths water. In this chapter, we'll discuss three simple biohacks for jump-starting a nutritional transformation, as well as one advanced technique you can use to improve your eating habits and provide your body with the best fuel possible.

Fat

When the months of spring start sliding by and summer's warmth and sunshine remind us of the approach of pool parties and beach excursions, many of us feel, not excited about the approaching season, but a paralyzing moment of panic. In order to drop those extra pounds left over from the holidays, we start thinking about dieting. There are literally thousands of fad diets, cleanses, and big-name diets that seem attractive at the onset, but these restrictive eating plans are only temporary fixes to a long-term problem. These temporary fixes are very difficult to maintain in the long term, and the only surefire way to improve physical health is to make lifestyle changes, not short-term adjustments.

You might be shocked to hear that the key to dramatic nutritional improvement is actually quite simple. Forget all of that complicated nutritional science for one minute, and make this easy phrase your mantra: Good Food, Good Fats. That's really all you need to know to change your health. Now, sure, there's a lot that goes into this mantra. It's important to avoid genetically modified organisms, meat products derived from caged animals, or meat products derived from animals that were fed inappropriate or unnatural diets. Chickens, for example, are evolutionarily accustomed to eating insects. Vegetarian-fed chickens, then, are unnatural, and therefore should be avoided.

When you choose foods to eat, try to consume foods that are as close to their natural, organic state as possible.

The "Good Foods" part of this nutritional mantra is easy to accept, but many people balk at the second part: Good Fats. We've been told, time and again, that fats are something to be avoided. If you want to lose that fat around your midsection, you should stop eating fats, right? Wrong. Good fats are key to a healthy diet. They make you feel fuller, happier, more productive, and more alert. They stabilize blood sugar levels to prevent that afternoon "crash" indicative of a high-carb diet.

What are good fats? Olive oil, nuts, wild-caught fish, fish oils, coconut oil, grass-fed butter, pastured egg yolks, pastured or heritage-raised pork, and other natural, healthy fats will not contribute to heart disease, raise your cholesterol levels, or make you fat. This is because they have the optimal balance of Omega-3s and Omega-6s. Fat consumption leads to a healthier body because our bodies are naturally intended to be fat burners, not carbohydrate burners!

Excessive carbohydrate consumption, especially the consumption of sugar, confuses the human body. The presence of so much fast-burning fuel overwhelms the body. Because it has no use for so many carbohydrates, it converts carbs into stores of fat, so it can use those stores later. The problem is, we keep delivering carbs to the body, encouraging it to create additional fat stores without ever giving it a reason to use the stores we already have.

What's the best fat to consume on a daily basis? MCT Oil, derived from coconuts, is made up of short- and medium-change triglycerides. These shorter triglyceride chains are immediately available for use by the human body. Consuming oils with shorter triglyceride chains turns us into lean, mean, fat-burning machines. The fat is used rather than stored, fat-soluble vitamins like A, D, E, and K are absorbed, ketones within the fats make our brains come alive, and we start to feel alive, vigorous, and highly focused.

Don't get overwhelmed by confusing nutritional science. This biohack is simple to understand and easy to remember. Eat foods that are as close to nature as possible. Increase healthy fat consumption. Eliminate excessive carb consumption by cutting out sugars. Remember: good food and good fats will create a sustainable, healthy diet.

Home

One of the biggest obstacles derailing healthy lifestyle changes amongst families is the habit of dining out. Dining out offers almost no control over nutrition, portion control, and ingredient quality. Cooking at home, on the other hand, is one of the best ways to improve overall nutrition.

We're super busy, though, and the idea of cooking dinner every night of the week is intimidating and exhausting. After a stressful work day, the prospect of picking up takeout rather than cooking a meal is enticing. There are companies, though, that can make the process of cooking at home infinitely easier.

For residents of New York City, check out Blue Apron. For those outside of the city or outside the country, a company called Hello Fresh is a great alternative. What do these companies offer? For around $10 per person, per meal, you'll receive a box that is filled with all of the ingredients needed to make a healthy, nutritious meal in just 30 minutes or less. The only ingredients you need to keep on hand are salt, pepper, and olive oil. Everything else comes neatly packaged in the box along with easy-to-follow cooking and preparation instructions. You can also keep the included recipe cards and reuse them in the future.

There is no planning, shopping, or advanced preparation required. In 30 minutes, with no required culinary knowledge or expertise, you'll be able to cook nutritious, delicious meals for the whole family. Let your local fast food restaurant fill someone else's stomach with nutritionally vacant foods. You and your family will be on the fast track to nutritional perfection.

Super

I'm reluctant to use the word "super" to describe foods in general. If you use basic, high quality ingredients to cook and prepare meals, all of those ingredients can have a super effect on your nutrition. However, it's important to mention that there are some foods that are simply packed with nutritional gold. Experts commonly refer to these foods as "superfoods," so it's terminology that we'll use in this section.

The very first, and often surprising, superfood is coffee. Coffee can have some adverse effects, like the caffeine jitters, and some people simply don't like the taste, but it's worth mentioning because of its nutritional benefits. Coffee is very simple: purchase coffee that is a single source, never a blend, and ideally purchase coffee that is grown in a high altitude environment. Higher altitude growing environments inhibit the growth of mold toxins.

Avocados are another excellent source of super nutrition. The fats in avocado are extraordinarily healthy, and this food can be used in a number of surprising ways. You can substitute avocado for other fats in cooking, baking, or even smoothie-making. The combination of protein and healthy fats makes avocado an excellent source of nutrition.

Greens are, of course, paramount in crafting a well-balanced diet. Most people don't get enough greens on a daily basis, and there's the added problem of inadequate vitamin absorption. Eating a super healthy green, like kale, is ineffective unless the right amount of fat is also consumed to dissolve fat-soluble vitamins. A good solution is wheatgrass powder. It is filled with vitamins, minerals, antioxidants, living enzymes, and chlorophyll. These ingredients detoxify the body and provide amazing levels of energy.

Cacao powder is a by-product of cocoa beans. When the beans are separated, the resultant products are cocoa butter and cacao powder. Cacao powder is high in iron and magnesium, and it acts as an antioxidant. Cultures around the world have historical records of cacao powder used as a health supplement. Legend says that Montezuma, the Aztec emperor, consumed fifty cups of hot cocoa each day! That doesn't sound too bad, does it?

Chia seeds are another important superfood. They are a significant part of Central American culture, and the famous book Born to Run references the Tarahumara tribe, which has used a mixture of chia seeds, water, and lime to make an energy-rich Chia Fresca beverage for centuries. Chia seeds are, in fact, the only vegan source of certain omega fatty acids, and the seeds also provide fiber and protein. Mixing chia seeds with water creates an anti-inflammatory, gut-healing gel that is great for individuals with digestive disorders.

Whey protein is another great superfood. It's important to choose a hydrolyzed whey protein concentrate or isolate. The hydrolyzing process essentially breaks down the whey molecules so they are more readily available to the body. Consumption of high quality whey protein concentrates will provide adequate levels of protein, energy, and much more.

Spirolina is a very interesting green. It provides an unbelievable array of minerals, vitamins, and antioxidants. There have been numerous studies performed showing how spirolina boosts brain function and acts as a powerful antioxidant, flushing toxins from the body. One of the reasons why supplementation is so important in a daily diet is that the average person's diet is simply not varied enough to provide adequate vitamin absorption. Additionally, over-farming and overuse of natural resources means that soil is often depleted of naturally occurring vitamins, and this vitamin depletion bleeds into the foods we eat. Spirolina is a great, natural vitamin supplement that will help round out a healthy diet.

When we think of superfoods, our minds quickly jump to healthy vegetables and superior fats. However, various spices are also important to consider. Turmeric, for example, is an incredibly nutritional and valuable spice. Individuals with chronic inflammatory issues or joint pain have reported dramatic relief from consuming turmeric. Cinnamon, too, is a potent superfood spice. This spice can increase circulation, it's antimicrobial and antibacterial, and it can even help with insulin regulation.

How can you use all of these super ingredients? Try making a delicious, fragrant, and powerful smoothie. Mix all of the ingredients above with almond milk or coconut milk and, perhaps, a little MTC oil. You'll have a filling, delicious, and powerfully nutritional breakfast beverage. If you crave some additional sweetness, try adding Xylitol, a sugar alcohol that our bodies don't digest. It's antibacterial and won't cause blood sugar spikes or other adverse effects.

In one beverage, you'll be consuming an amazing assortment of mega-healthy superfoods that will totally transform your health and jumpstart your day.

Advanced

If you're ready to take your nutritional journey to the next level, fasting is a great process to try. Here, we are not talking about general fasting for an indefinite period of time. Rather, we're referring to intermittent fasting: the regular pattern of alternating between food consumption and food abstention. Intermittent fasts come in all shapes and sizes. Some choose to eat for five days and fast for two days. Others alternate between a day of eating and a day of fasting.

Regardless of the specific eating and fasting time periods, there is an abundance of scientific research that supports the benefits of intermittent fasting. Generally speaking, fasting regulates hormone levels, changes the body's metabolism to encourage fat burning, and even changes our reaction to food, making eating a more fulfilling and pleasurable experience.

Ancestrally speaking, it's likely that our ancient relatives were unable to eat at every meal. With no agriculture or supermarkets, food was consumed when it was available, and the body was required to continue surviving and thriving, even when food was nowhere to be found. The human body, then, has adapted to an intermittent fasting lifestyle.

Here's an easy method for intermittent fasting: skip breakfast on a daily basis. There's that old adage that tells us breakfast is the most important meal of the day, but this is actually misleading. The first meal you eat is the most important meal of the day, but eating that meal within an hour of waking up may not be the best practice for overall health. It can be stressful to try to cram a meal into a fast-paced morning. Thinking about food during the first half of the day can create unnecessary stress, so why not push that meal back until lunchtime?

To get started with intermittent fasting, try this: between the hours of noon and 8:00 p.m., eat as much as you need to feel full. For the rest of the day, abstain completely from food. Try this for a few weeks, and see how you feel. You may be surprised by the results.

FIVE

supplements

As I mentioned in an earlier chapter, supplementation is an important part of overall nutrition. The sad truth is that our environment, agricultural processes, and average daily diets have changed dramatically in just a few decades. Aggressive farming practices have robbed the soil of important nutrients, which means that vegetables and fruits are lacking many of the nutrients our bodies need to survive. The types of foods that we consume, too, have changed over the years. Instead of consuming a wide variety of different food items, people today often subsist on a more narrow selection of foods. This reduces our consumption of nutrients and can leave the body lacking a few key elements.

There is a solution to reduced nutrient and vitamin availability, however. Supplementing our diets with natural, powerful sources of healthy nutrients will make up for any dietary gaps or shortcomings. There are thousands of supplements available on the market, though, and choosing the most important can be a challenge. In this chapter, we will discuss a few of the most beneficial supplements by choosing nutritional sources from the sea, land, and air.

Sea

Krill are tiny crustaceans, similar to shrimp, found in the North Atlantic, and these tiny organisms are virtually the only things that massive hump-back whales eat. The enormous whales consume tons of krill in a single day, deriving almost all of their nutrients from the pinprick-sized creatures. We, too, can benefit from the oil derived from krill.

Krill oil is actually better absorbed than fish oil by the human body, and it contains both EPA and DHA, the most important nutrients in fish oils. Studies have even shown that krill oil has forty times the antioxidizing power of other fish oils. This is just the tip of the iceberg, however.

C-Reactive Protein is one of the leading contributors to dangerous in-flammation in the human body, inflammation that can lead to debilitating diseases like Crohn's disease. There is currently a 100% scientific consensus on the ability of krill oil to reduce the levels of C-reactive protein in the human body. Studies have also shown that individuals struggling to reduce LDL cholesterol levels through typical means were able to see a dramatic reduction in this harmful cholesterol, as well as an increase in healthy HDL cholesterol, when supplementing their diets with krill oil. Krill oil may also help to improve brain function, reduce arthritis symptoms, regulate insulin, and accomplish many other feats in the human body. Amazingly, it has no adverse side effects.

A daily krill oil supplement will have dramatic, positive effects on your overall health and nutrition levels.

Land

When examining supplements derived from land organisms, probiotics have, perhaps, the most profound and powerful effect on human health. Unfortunately, most of us really lack a good balance of bacterial organisms in our bodies. The overuse of sanitizers and cleansers, the lack of exposure to the natural environment, and the periodic administration of powerful antibiotics have all eliminated healthy, necessary bacteria from our digestive systems.

GNC's Ultra 50 Probiotic Complex is a great supplement to replace these healthy bacteria. Each capsule contains 50 billion health bacterial organisms. Taking a probiotic supplement, rather than simply relying on foods like yogurt to increase probiotic populations in the body, is important because stomach acids kill the vast majority of probiotic organisms before they can reach the intestines. A probiotic pill is equipped with a coating to resist stomach acid and deliver probiotics where they are needed the most.

Look for supplements that contain multiple probiotic strains, like Lactobacillus acidophilus, Bifidobacterium bifidum, and Bifidobacterium lactis. Another important ingredient in probiotic supplements is Fructoligosaccharides: a sugar product that feeds the probiotic organisms, encouraging them to grow and thrive in your digestive tract. Interestingly enough, this sugar is found naturally in human breast milk, which may be a contributing factor to health disorders in babies fed formula rather than breast milk. In fact, my own mother was unable to breastfeed after giving birth to me, and I suffered from both eczema and Crohn's disease: two inflammatory illnesses.

Probiotics help with everything from colic to Irritable Bowel Syndrome, yeast infections to urinary tract infections, and even bad breath and excessive stress levels. Unless you are consuming massive amounts of fermented foods like miso, sauerkraut, kimchi, or yogurt, a probiotic supplement is a necessity.

Sky

I can confidently say that most people taking my course, listening to my lectures, or even reading this manuscript have a Vitamin D deficiency. It's just an inevitable truth. Vitamin D deficiencies are a by-product of our modern lives. We work inside. We cover our bodies with clothing year-round. We don't enough fat, which is necessary for the absorption of Vitamin D. All of these factors contribute to low Vitamin D levels in the body.

Vitamin D has a myriad of positive effects on the human body, including a reduced risk for bone breaks, reduced cardiovascular disease risk, and even a reduction in the risk of cancer. New studies have shown that there is a correlation between the presence of cancer and reduced Vitamin D levels.

An important trick to know about Vitamin D supplementation is when to take it. Vitamin D should always be consumed in the morning. This vitamin is inversely related to melatonin, a substance in the body that encourages sleepiness. If you take Vitamin D at night, it can impede the production of melatonin, causing restlessness and insomnia. Taking it in the morning may actually improve your sleep quality because of its inverse relationship with melatonin.

Advanced

Krill oil, probiotics, and Vitamin D are three of the most basic supplements that offer universal benefits to people. Generally speaking, everyone could stand to consume more of these essential nutrients on a daily basis. In this advanced section, though, I'm going to mention a supplement that I consider an advanced biohack: Creatine.

Creatine is a supplement worth experimenting with. You may have heard of this supplement in connection with athletes or bodybuilders because of its performance-enhancing effects. The truth is, though, that creatine is a natural supplement; it's produced naturally in the human body, and every body uses creatine. Because of this, creatine is one of the most studied and researched supplements in the world, and the majority of the findings reveal this to be a positive supplement with minimal side effects. One side effect worth mentioning is water retention, which can lead to temporary weight gain. With regular use, as the body's hydration levels regulate, however, this effect will subside.

More important than improving hydration, however, is creatine's ability to increase the power output of the body. This is especially helpful for weight lifting, as your muscles will be able to lift heavier weights, leading to increased muscle mass. Creatine also supports the building of lean mass in the body, and may increase the body's VO2 max, which is the body's ability to process oxygen.

With so many positive effects, it is worth your time to examine creatine's effects on your own body. You might discover that this supplement helps you with athletic performance, muscle building, or performance-enhancing hydration.

SIX
productivity

So far in this course, we've discussed a wide assortment of biohacks that are directly related to improving physical health. Boosting fitness levels, improving sleep habits, developing positive nutritional habits, and supplementing the diet are all great biohacks that can have dramatic effects on the physical body. Improving physical health is directly related to mental and spiritual health, but there are other important factors to consider when biohacking your life from top to bottom.

One great way to boost your mental health is to focus on improving productivity. I would be surprised to find anyone who couldn't admit that productivity enhancement would powerfully improve his or her daily life. Let's face it: productivity is a challenge, especially in today's modern world. Our focus is split a thousand different ways, we're bombarded with tasks and deadlines that need to be completed, and we're surrounded by distractions that are trying to keep us from accomplishing what needs to be done.

In this chapter, we'll discuss three basic biohacks for improving productivity, including optimization, automation, and outsourcing. Then, we'll take a look at an advanced biohack to take your productivity journey to the next level.

Optimize

Let's start with optimizing your daily life. One of the major problems destroying productivity is the overwhelming number of tasks, chores, ideas, and thoughts that run through our mind throughout the day. You could solve this problem by covering your walls with Post-It notes, but this impractical and chaotic.

What we need is a tool that allows us to organize and optimize our daily lives, and we need to know how best to use that tool to generate increased productivity. One great note-taking application with unlimited power is Evernote. With this software, you can make notes that consist of text, web pages, photos, or audio clips and sync these notes amongst all of your devices, including smart phones, desktop computers, laptops, and tablets.

Evernote is simple, intuitive, and incredibly powerful. The key to getting the most use out of this program is to overuse it. If there is an idea in your head, you need to get it out of your head and get it onto Evernote. Your brain has a capacity, and too many ideas and thoughts floating around in there can lead to chaos and clutter. You don't need to know if the idea is relevant, worth preserving, or beneficial whatsoever. When you place the idea into Evernote, you'll know that it's safe and there for examining and evaluating at a future time.

Evernote allows you to let go, move on, and work on the next task. It's also a learning program. As you begin to clip articles, videos, and other content from the web, Evernote starts learning what interests you. It begins to display notes that are relevant to you and to the task you are currently working on.

For example, if you're browsing the Internet and you clip an interesting blog post to your Evernote collection, the software will display notes that are relevant or connected to the blog post you've just clipped. These notes might be from a year ago, a few months ago, or even a day before.

At the time, you may not have known why those notes were relevant, but now Evernote displays them in conjunction with one another, and you've essentially pulled information from your past to display a complete, relevant thought.

You can also use Evernote to keep track of your everyday tasks. All of the minute details and "microsteps" required to get you through the day or to complete larger tasks can be evaluated in a highly organized way. As you evaluate your daily routine, you can begin to optimize that routine. Optimization leads to automation, and automation leads to outsourcing. This one program can take a hectic, jam-packed day of tasks and duties and turn it into a streamlined, efficient process.

Use Evernote as your external brain, and start focusing on what's really important.

Automate

If there's one productivity tool that everyone should be using, it's Follow-Up.cc. This is a very basic service that can be used in some amazing and advanced way. Essentially, this is an automated follow-up email service that can be used from any platform or any browser. There is no longer any reason to create calendar events to remind you to follow-up with email recipients. With FollowUp.cc, you can use the CC or BCC fields in the email entry field to schedule an automated reminder to follow up with that individual.

Choosing the timeframe for the follow-up is simple. In order to schedule an email reminder to be delivered to your inbox in one week, just type 1week@followup.cc into the CC or BCC section of the email. You can put calendar dates, days of the weeks, or hour durations into the email, so the customization options are endless. Entering the delay date into the CC field will deliver the same email to both you and the original recipient at the specified time. Entering the date into the BCC field will deliver the reminder only to you, the sender.

FollowUp.cc also has a brilliant snooze functionality. When you receive the reminder email from FollowUp.cc, you can click on several different links to "snooze" the email and receive it at a later date. Choose minutes, hours, days, weeks, or even a specific day of the week to deal with the email at a later time.

The way this program becomes so powerful is when it allows you to achieve "Inbox Zero." Your email inbox should be a place of action. There are only three things you can do with an email: delete it when the subject is completed, act on it when the subject can be dealt with immediately, or defer it to a more appropriate time. Don't be mistaken; deferring and procrastinating are not the same thing. Procrastination is ignoring a task simply because you don't want to deal with it. Deferring tasks is putting them off to a time where you can deal with the task in a more appropriate way.

FollowUp.cc allows you to defer the appropriate emails to clean up your inbox and remove clutter. More importantly, though, it ensures that nothing important slips through the cracks ever again. If you meet a valuable contact and send an email inviting the contact to meet over coffee in the future, FollowUp.cc will allow you to set a reminder to reconnect, or follow up, with that individual at the appropriate time.

When you use this impressive program, sending an email means you don't have to think about a task or responsibility again. You don't have to manage calendars or correspondence in your head. When it's time to deal with the task again, you'll receive an email. It's a simple to-do list that will permanently improve your productivity.

Outsource

Now, let's spend some time talking about outsourcing. Outsourcing is something that many people feel belongs only in a large corporation. Sometimes, we even have a negative view of outsourcing. Everyone has experienced the frustration of calling a business's customer service hotline only to discover that the entire customer service department has been outsourced to a foreign country.

Outsourcing is not a large-scale enterprise that is only appropriate for large-scale businesses. A single individual can benefit from outsourcing. Think, for a minute, of all the tiny, tedious tasks that you complete in a single day. Tasks like making restaurant reservations, buying groceries, running errands, performing Internet searches, managing accounts and billing, and even calling frustrating customer service hotlines can all be outsourced and performed by another individual or company.

FancyHands is the online organization I use for all my outsourcing needs. I simply create a message, sometimes attach a photo to further explain my query or need, and send the request off to be handled by their professionals. Then, I move on to a completely different task. While I am focused elsewhere, FancyHands is taking care of my task or problem for me. I'm alerted when the task is completed, and with very little effort I have immediately saved time.

Time is time. Any time that you save by outsourcing tasks is time that you can use for other purposes. It may take awhile to train yourself to outsource even the simplest of tasks to a business like FancyHands, but the more frequently you can outsource tasks the more deposits you are making into your available time bank.

Advanced

In order to further improve my own productivity and hopefully help boost productivity in others, I started developing a system called Less Doing: doing less but getting more. My solution is all about optimizing, automating, and outsourcing everything in life to make things easier.

Optimization involves a lot of quantified self data collection, the creation of proper goals, and the development of achievable milestones. My work with optimization began to develop into a coaching business framework. Now, I work with a variety of individuals with issues ranging from health to business to relationships. My goal, then, is to work with clients to make them better at just about anything they set their minds to.

I had a client who wanted to reduce his running mile time from nine and a half minutes to seven minutes in 90 days. We achieved his goal in 66 days. Another client provided me with a laundry list of 25 tasks he hoped to accomplish that consisted of goals like outsourcing an assistant position and even learning the process of lucid dreaming. Everyone has something they want to accomplish. Less Doing is the process I use to turn goals into achievements.

By looking at these abstract goals from a removed position, I am able to provide fresh perspective. That perspective is often all that is necessary to move forward and achieve a goal. If you're interested in taking your productivity to the next level, I invite you to check out Less Doing and let me help you remove obstacles, begin a goal-seeking journey, and cross milestones off your to-do list, once and for all.

SEVEN
tracking

If you've ever kept a journal, you know what an incredibly effective and interesting tool it can be for self-discovery. Many people keep journals or diaries as children or young adults, and it can be fascinating to read back over these journals after months or even years have passed.

Journaling is just one aspect of a self-discovery process known as tracking. Tracking involves keeping a record of activities, goals, accomplishments, setbacks, moods, emotions, and other important self-related data. With this data, self-improvement becomes a more effective process. Interpreting this data allows us to identify strengths and weaknesses, improve certain aspects of our lives, and more easily reach goals and milestones.

This chapter discusses some ways to biohack the tracking process, using powerful and simple tools like websites and software to create a record of your daily life.

Input

Whether we're talking about granular events like sent emails or completed tasks or evaluating larger things like psychological well-being or general feelings about a specific day, self-tracking through regular input is incredibly important.

IDoneThis.com is an incredibly simple and powerful tool. Basically, every night you will receive an email around 6:00 p.m. asking you what you accomplished in the day. All that is required of you, then, is to write back and say what you've done. This could be an accomplishment at work, a failure or setback, a personal achievement, anything.

It's easy, in the midst of a busy day, to focus on the negative rather than acknowledging the many accomplishments and steps forward that we achieved. Taking 30 seconds at the end of the day to think, "What did I get done today?" is a powerful habit in and of itself. IDoneThis.com, though, doesn't stop there.

When you use this site on a regular basis, your nightly email will start to change. In addition to being prompted to discuss your daily achievements, IDoneThis.com will start reminding you of past achievements. You might get a reminder about what was achieved the day before, the week before, or even several months before.

These reminders, remarkably, are not randomized. IDoneThis uses a proprietary algorithm to display relevant achievements when you need to see them most. The process is nothing short of miraculous. I cannot tell you how many times I've had what I thought was a bad day only to be reminded by IDoneThis of a massive achievement I'd made weeks before.

This service is also available for teams, which is great for team motivation and collective monitoring of goal accomplishment. There is a personal calendar attribute where you can visit any and all past days to review accomplishments and monitor goal achievement progress. There is also an amazing visual portal on your dashboard that creates a word cloud showing you common words, concepts, and ideas that recur regularly in your IDoneThis responses.

Output

When I teach my seminars in person, I always pose this challenge: "Raise your hands really quickly if you can tell me, without thinking about it, what you had for breakfast this morning." Usually, about 90% of the people in the room put their hands in the air. My next challenge is a little more difficult: "Raise your hands if you can tell me, without thinking about it, how many emails you sent last Tuesday." The number of hands is almost always zero.

What's the point, you might wonder, of remembering how many emails you sent on an arbitrary day? If you can track this output, and monitor or assess the data, you might find something actionable that could improve your productivity.

RescueTime.com is an application that sits in the background of your computer and watches your daily activity. It will tell you how much time you are spending on various website, in different applications, and even in different documents. You can use this data to identify time-wasting websites that are distracting you from completing important tasks. You can set goals for yourself to accomplish various tasks in a certain time frame.

Another useful feature is the weekly summary emails that quickly show you where you are spending most of your time, both on and off the computer. RescueTime can even keep track of time spent away from the computer, so you can monitor how much time you spend at the gym, in your vehicle, running errands, etc.

One of the most useful features, though, is the focus feature. You can engage this feature to temporarily block all of your personal timewasting websites for a specified period of time. So, if you have trouble with drifting onto Twitter when trying to avoid an important task, you can block Twitter for thirty minutes to encourage focus and goal accomplishment.

This leads us to an interesting and effective biohack tangent called the Pomodoro Technique. Essentially, this technique is based on the idea that work should be completed in 25 minute segments, with four to five minutes of rest in between. This is based on the concept that our brain works in sprints, rather than marathons. It's also useful for identifying how long it takes to complete various tasks. For example, if you have to make a PowerPoint presentation for work, you begin by writing down the name and nature of the task on a piece of paper.

Next, set your timer for 25 minutes and begin working on the task. When the timer rings, stop working and take a break. Mark an "X" on the paper. This represents one spurt of productivity. When the task is complete, you can count the number of X's to determine how long it takes for you to complete a PowerPoint presentation.

RescueTime will help you monitor your productivity throughout the day or throughout the week. You can identify low-productivity hours during the day to identify and fix potential problems. The possibilities are endless, and RescueTime requires no active input on your part. Simple run the program in the background and watch the data roll in.

Self

Tracking your productivity, activities, and goals is very important, but tracking your actual health is also crucial. InsideTracker.com is a helpful website that allows you to submit your own blood and view a comprehensive analysis of your bloodwork results. You may wonder, "Why can't I just leave this process to my physician?" The truth is, many doctors only request the bare minimum of available tests, so the picture of your health that you get from your doctor may be incomplete. More importantly, you won't receive the same access when you rely on your doctor. Inside-Tracker gives you a visual record of your bloodwork, so you can compare your results over time and monitor health and progress.

InsideTracker's bloodwork is astoundingly comprehensive. You can view data regarding your energy and metabolism, including levels of glucose, cholesterol, LDL, HDL, and triglycerides. You'll see information about strength and endurance, bone and muscle health, brain and body health, and even performance.

Taking your blood is simple. InsideTracker provides you with all the materials you need. All that is required is a few drops collected from a fingertip prick. You apply the blood to a sterile slide that InsideTracker provides, send the blood in the mail, and in a short time log in to view your results.

This type of tracking can be invaluable, and you can customize the process to fit your specific needs. For example, imagine that you want to monitor your own hormone levels over the course of the next ten years. Checking your testosterone levels now will help you identify ailing T levels in the future. Knowing the real-time status of your body's health is empowering and extraordinarily valuable.

Advanced

In this advanced section, I'm going to show you the wide array of products and services that I use on a regular basis to monitor and track just about everything. With the products and services mentioned in this section, you will have everything you need to fully monitor your physical, mental, and emotional health. There are several things to consider in this advanced section, and it's not important to invest in all of them at once or even all of them ever. Choose the tracking tools that you think will benefit you most.

The following tools are ranked from the least invasive and easiest to use to the most invasive and challenging to use:

- Withings Body Scale: Checks your weight, resting heart rate, body fat, and even the air quality in the room. This scale has Wi-Fi capabilities, so it will automatically upload this information, which makes it easy to track your data over time.
- Basis Activity Monitor: There are tons of fitness and activity monitors available, but in my opinion the Basis brand is the best of the best. This product goes way beyond motion sensing capabilities; it has skin

temperature sensors, sweat sensors, and other features to evaluate how much energy your burning and how it's affecting you.

- Amigo Wristband: This product measures heart rate, and it also measures hundreds of activities automatically. It can tell the difference between jumping jacks, spin cycling, running, road biking, and much more.
- RescueTime: We've covered this in a previous section. This is, in my opinion, the best tool for monitoring activity on your computer.
- RunKeeper: It's advertised as a personal trainer in your pocket, and that's truly what it is. You can install this application directly to your smartphone. As you run, the app will track your pace and distance, deliver prompts into your ears while you're listening to music, and integrates social media to allow friends to track your run live and offer encouragement.
- Gym Hero: RunKeeper actually syncs and works in conjunction with this application. This is a great app for tracking workouts, exercises, weights, sets and reps, and much more. Tracking your workouts in this way will help you identify weak areas and develop a more focused workout routine.
- Sleep Cycle: We've covered sleep before, but Sleep Cycle is an iPhone app that monitors the vibrations in your bed during the night to determine your sleep cycles. Our bodies are fairly still during deep sleep, so Sleep Cycle can tell you how much deep sleep you're getting, how many full sleep cycles you complete in a night, and it even has an alarm function that will attempt to wake you during the lightest sleep stage.
- Thryve: There are thousands of food tracking apps available, but I like Thryve for a very simple reason. It's the only one that offers the option to track how you feel. This is important because many people don't make the connection between the foods they are eating and the way they are feeling. That connection is easily made with Thryve.
- MoodScope: Tracking mood is a subjective process in many ways, but it can be very helpful if done regularly. People who track their moods may be able to overcome depression symptoms, identify their best and most productive times of day, and understand how their mood is affected by season, diet, and environment.
- Cardiio.com: If you just want to track your heart rate, Cardiio.com is

such a cool app. If nothing else, simply using the app is a lot of fun. It uses the iPhone's camera to detect subtle color changes in the skin of your face. Using that information, it can calculate your heart rate. You can determine your resting heart rate, track your rate over time, and work on lowering your heart rate as you get in shape.

- Withings: For blood pressure monitoring, the Withings blood pressure cuff is simple and effective. Simply slide the cuff on your arm, plug it into your iPhone, and it automatically determines your blood pressure. A nice feature is the integration between multiple Withings products, making data easy to track.
- Stress Check: This app is fairly basic. Using heart rate technology, the application takes your heart rate and assigns you a number between 1 and 100. This number is how stressed you are. You may feel very relaxed or stressed, but this app helps to identify if something else is going on. The app can be used to customize workout routines based on current stress levels or indicate when you might benefit from a period of meditation or relaxation, say, before that big meeting in an hour.
- Mentor: This is an app that helps you create habits and, more importantly, reach your goals. Whether you want to run a marathon, read more frequently, or just stop biting your nails, Mentor will help you get there.
- Mint: This is a great app for tracking finances. Mint uses your bank account information to monitor your spending habits, assist with budget creation, alert you to overspending, and even provide you with customized sales and discount opportunities based on your spending tastes.
- Tinke: This is basically a wellness monitor; it allows you to check your heart rate variability, your pulse, the oxygen in your blood, and a few other metrics. It's a little more advanced than some of the other sensors on the market, and it offers a more comprehensive way to measure overall health.
- Scanadu: This device is being called the closest thing to a tricorder ever created. The Scanadu Scout, as well as the Scanaflow, will allow you to test and monitor metrics like temperature, heart rate, ECG, heart rate variability, pulse wave transit time, urine analysis, stress, and more. This is a lot of information to measure without requiring a

professional, and it will further help you identify stress factors, environmental factors, and other key health influences.

- AliveCor: If you want to get serious about your heart, AliveCor has created an FDA-approved heart monitor that provides the real sonogram. The app provides an authentic electrocardiogram display, which makes it exceptionally beneficial for people who've had heart problems in the past.

- Brain Turk: We've mentioned Brain Turk before. This is another way of tracking the way your cognitive functions are working. You can use the app as a tracking device to determine if and how environment, foods, sleep habits, and other factors affect your thinking processes.

- uBiome: This lets you test the micro-biome of your body. Basically, this means testing your poop, but you can also test your nasal passages, mouth, ears, and genitals to get an overall picture of your micro-biome and the bacteria that make up your body. This is not yet a diagnostic tool, but you can learn a lot about your bodily functions and health by identifying the populations of bacteria catching a ride inside your body.

- InsideTracker: As mentioned above, this is a great self-test tool that allows you to view highly specific and comprehensive bloodwork analysis. There are a couple dozen different biomarkers offered, and you can monitor changes in your blood over time.

- 23andMe: This is a genetic testing company. You provide a vial of saliva, and 23andMe will test for over 240 health conditions and traits as well as 40 inherited conditions. You can even find out about your ancestry. The information is updated regularly, so you'll receive email updates when new genetic information becomes available.

- Dexcom: This is definitely the most hardcore. The Dexcom G4 is a wireless, continuous glucose monitor. Essentially, this device is implanted in your side. It is not comfortable, but if you are diabetic or you simply want to see how certain meals or activities affect your blood glucose levels on a constant basis, this is the best way to do just that.

- TicTrac: This is, essentially, data analysis for data idiots. I love tracking data, but I certainly don't consider myself a data analysis specialist. That's why TicTrac is so helpful. You can enter data from several different sources, including exercise and workout data, spreadsheets, heart rate monitors, and create visual correlations that will help you see what the data means. Based on your own experiments and your own desires, you can determine how X affects Y, and that's the best way to make real changes.

EIGHT

recovery

O ur lives are hectic. Our schedules are chaotic. Our lives are demanding. Our bodies undergo massive amounts of stress and strain each and every day. Starting a regular workout routine can be a great way to alleviate stress while simultaneously improving overall health and wellness, but there is always a risk of sustaining a strain injury during a workout.

Whether you're injured or just exhausted from a regular day, one thing that is missing from most people's lives is adequate rest, recovery, recuperation, and rejuvenation. This chapter is all about recovery biohacks that will rejuvenate the body, promote healing, and lead to a healthier, happier life.

Hot and Cold

One of the simplest things you can do to aid in workout recovery or simply shed the stressed of a tough day is Contrast Hydrotherapy. That's a technical name that's used to describe a relatively simple process. Basically, we're talking about alternating hot and cold temperatures on your body. You can do this through immersions in a bath or temperature fluctuations in a sauna, but the easiest way to do it is in a shower.

The benefits of Contrast Hydrotherapy are pretty numerous, but basically the process stimulates blood flow, helps to reduce swelling, and helps to relax tissue and muscle. As an added side benefit, there is evidence to show that you can achieve cold thermogenesis, which is the act of your body burning brown adipose fat tissue. When your body is exposed to cold temperatures, it burns this tissue to keep warm, and you end up burning calories and using up fat stores.

The simplest way to do a contrast shower is very similar to the Tabata exercise process we discussed in the Fitness section of this manuscript. In the shower, start with 20 seconds of cold water. The water shouldn't be freezing because this can stress the body, but it should be uncomfortably cold. These 20 seconds of cold water are followed by 10 seconds of warm water. The greatest possible difference between the two temperatures will yield the best effect, but temperatures that are too extreme will cause unnecessary stress. Perform this pattern of alternating temperatures 10 times, for a total time of 5 minutes. You can add this Contrast Hydrotherapy method to the end of your normal shower. It's a great way to jumpstart your recovery process.

Compress

Anyone who has ever participated in an endurance sport, long-distance running, or a Triathlon-type event knows about compression tights, but for those of you who don't it's a pretty basic concept. These tights are worn after a long workout or even a long day of continued standing. The tights compress your muscles in a specific, optimized way to maintain circulation and recovery. The feeling is akin to fifty hands deeply massaging your muscles as you move. When you first try them on, they will feel oddly tight and slightly restrictive, and this is completely normal.

You can purchase calf socks or compression shorts, but I personally recommend the full tights that stretch from ankle to stomach. You can wear these compression tights after a workout, while sitting on the plane, or even while you sleep.

110% is a company that manufactures a special pair of compression tights that contain ice packs that work in conjunction with the compression material. Not only will you get the benefit of optimized compression over your muscles, but you'll also be able to apply soothing cold temperatures to reduce inflammation and stimulate cold thermogenesis.

You'll learn to love these tights. They become very comfortable, and you can wear them for prolonged periods of time to get maximum benefit.

Earth

For those of you not familiar with the concept of "Earthing," you may find this just a little bit weird to begin with, but I assure you that this concept is supported by science and research. Earthing is based on the idea that we are losing touch with our connection to the earth and its natural resources. By wearing shoes and socks, living in sophisticated homes, and driving vehicles rather than walking, we're missing out on valuable negative ions that enter our bodies through direct skin-to-earth contact and assist with detoxification and rejuvenation.

If that sounds a little out there, consider the way you feel after a long walk on the beach or after running your feet through soft, fragrant dirt. There is something tactile, mental, spiritual, and even physical that happens when our bodies are connected with the earth.

Earthing is an attempt to reestablish that lost connection. There are wristbands, desk mats, and other products available, but the simplest method is with an Earthing sheet. This sheet goes over your bed and creates a pathway between the earth and your body, allowing for the exchange of potent ions. There is no electrification or charge exchange happening with this sheet. You simply sleep on the Earthing sheets like you would any normal bed sheet, and you will experience more restful sleep, boosted recovery, and whole-body rejuvenation.

I know, it sounds far-fetched and a little strange. Try one for yourself, and see if you experience the transformative powers of Earthing. I think you will.

Advanced

In the advanced section of Recovery, I'd like to discuss a powerfully effective technique known as electrical stimulation. Electrical muscular stimulation is not a new technology by any means. Physical therapists use it because it helps with strengthening and rehabilitation because, essentially, what it's doing is contracting and relaxing your muscles for you. Sometimes, electrical stimulation can actually work your muscles harder and more intensely than you could do without assistance, even if you contracted your muscles as tightly as possible.

This assisted contraction and relaxation works the muscles rapidly and helps to flush out the accumulation of lactic acid. You can also use electrical muscular stimulation for training. For instance, if you are training to improve your squat, you can place stimulation pads on your thigh muscles to contract those muscles at an accelerated rate. Over time, your muscles will develop a "memory" of this motion. When you head to the gym and heft a squat bar in a "real" workout setting, your muscles will recall what it feels like to expand and contract the critical thigh muscles, and you'll find that you're able to lift heavier and faster during a workout.

There are lots of different electrical stimulation units available, but I'm personally a fan of Slendertone's products. They can be purchased for under $75, which makes them a great value. They don't have a lot of the special features that other products come with, but it's a quality unit that will help with recovery. This is a great way to experiment with electrical muscular stimulation to determine if this biohack works for you.

If you're looking for the "Cadillac" quality product, the Compex MI-Sport, priced at well over $1000, comes with different modes such as warm-up, recovery, and conditioning, so you can dial in the program you want to get the most out of the product.

Either way, the product basically utilizes the same basic mechanism.

Electrical muscular stimulation is a great biohack that will help you shorten recovery time, increase lean muscle mass, and improve overall performance.

ADVANCED

the next level

I really hope you've enjoyed this course as an introduction to biohacking. Biohacking is a personal passion of mine, and it's a part of me that constantly strives to improve aspects of my life in every possible way. That passion has grown and developed into a mission to show others the amazing benefits of biohacking and health optimization.

While this introductory course provided a few basic biohacking techniques as well as a handful of advanced techniques to help you take your biohacking to the next level, there is certainly more information out there to learn. You might be thinking right now of a specific health condition that is plaguing you or a specific goal that you have yet to achieve. Whether you're struggling with diabetes or obesity or the goal is something like better cognition, better memory, or the protection from hereditary illnesses, there is information available for you to absorb and implement.

I've shown you a lot of different ways to test yourself and gather data on yourself, and even if you are not a "data person," my theory is that collecting enough data will eventually open up a pathway to self-discovery. At some point in your journey, you will discover an area of weakness, a potential for improvement, or a health effect that was previously unknown or unexplored in your life. When you identify these areas of interest, using your data collection, there are many great resources available to help you develop new biohacking techniques and new ways to improve.

PubMed.gov is a clearinghouse for all sorts of medical studies. They have legitimacy, and you can read the abstracts and evaluate the science and research for yourself. This will help you make informed decisions about questions you might currently have. Is saturated fat really bad for you? Does this particular medication cause inflammation? You can search any number of topics and vastly expand your knowledge base.

Another great resource is Examine.com. Essentially, this site takes the studies from PubMed, groups them together, and creates a user-friendly, searchable list that will help you navigate the wealth of information available. One great feature is the Health Goals section, where you can browse different topics and evaluate different studies that show what kinds of compounds help with a particular condition. Many of the illnesses and conditions you'll find have an inflammatory component to them, and even if you don't have any sort of chronic illness, everybody deals with inflammation on some level. We can all afford to evaluate anti-inflammatory foods, supplements, habits, and environmental changes to some extent.

With Examine.com, you can read about a particular compound, like fish oil, and see what effect it has had in scientific studies on test subjects. Then, you can use your tracking biohacking skills to test that compound's effect in your own life. These resources empower you to personalize biohacking. Every body is different, and what works for you may not work for others. Above all, the quest for knowledge will inspire you and encourage you to keep improving your body, your health, your mental capacities, your productivity and goal journeys, and many other areas of wellness.

Finally, I'd like to end by saying that I do work with people who have illnesses or simply wish to perform better. Through LessDoing.com,

I've been able to do that more efficiently and more effectively. I created LessDoing as a method of dealing with stress as a direct result of a chronic disease that I suffered with: Crohn's Disease. Now, I've been pain free and medicine free for four years.

I encourage you to check out the website, sign up for the newsletter, and read a few blog posts to see if anything interests you. I always try to create new, valuable, interesting content about productivity, wellness, and overall health. I believe that our goal-achieving potential is stronger when we work together, and I invite you to partner with me on a quest for whole body, whole mind vitality.

Thank you again, and stay tuned for further updates!

RESOURCES

I've mentioned a lot of websites, smartphone applications, and brand-name products in this book. While you don't need to rush out and purchase everything I've referenced, I stand by these products and services and believe they offer great value to anyone interested in improving health through biohacking techniques. For your future reference, I've included a list of helpful sites, products, and apps for you to consult as you begin your biohacking journey.

Websites:

- BrainTurk.com
- BrainScape.com
- Onnit.com
- Sleepyti.me
- BlueApron.com
- HelloFresh.com
- Evernote.com
- FollowUp.cc
- FancyHands.com
- IDoneThis.com
- RescueTime.com
- InsideTracker.com
- MoodScope.com
- Cardiio.com
- 23andMe.com
- TicTrac.com
- PubMed.gov
- Examine.com

Products:

- Remee Sleep Mask
- GNC Ultra50
- Withings Body Scale
- Basis Activity Monitor
- Amigo Wristband
- Withings BP Cuff
- Tinke
- Scanadu
- AliveCor
- uBiome
- Dexcom
- Slendertone
- Compex MI-Sport

Apps:

- Yoga Studio
- Stress Doctor
- Evernote
- Run Keeper
- Gym Hero
- Sleep Cycle
- Thryve
- Stress Check
- Mentor
- Mint

Be sure to check out my site, LessDoing.com, for more information about helpful products, services, websites, and applications. Best of luck to you on your biohacking journey!

Printed in Great Britain
by Amazon

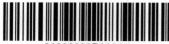